SMOOTHIES FOR DIVERTICULITIS

Boost Your Immune System, Soothe Your Gut: Delicious Smoothies for Diverticulitis and Overall Digestive Wellness

SELENA LEONARD

Table of Contents

INTRODUCTION 12

Dive into Digestive Wellness: A Smooth Path to Managing Diverticulitis 12

A Note from Selena Leonard: 14

Chapter 1: 16

Demystifying Diverticulitis: Symptoms, Causes, and Management Strategies 16

1.1 What is Diverticulitis? 16

1.2 Recognizing the Signs and Symptoms: 17

1.3 Understanding the Triggers and Risk Factors: 18

1.4 Conventional Treatment Approaches: 19

Chapter 2: 22

The Power of Smoothies: Benefits for Digestion and Overall Health 22

2.1 Advantages of Smoothies for Individuals with Diverticulitis 22

2.2 Choosing the Right Ingredients: Fiber, Nutrients, and Antioxidants: 25

2.3 Building a Balanced and Delicious Smoothie Base:25

2.4 Tips for Perfecting Texture and Flavor:.................. 26

Chapter 3:... 28

Soothing Smoothies for Flare-Up Relief and Gut Calming

.... 28

Ginger Green Glory (Serves 1)................................. 28

Tropical Calming (Serves 1)..................................... 31

Mellow Mango Magic (Serves 1) 31

Cooling Cucumber Comfort (Serves 1) 32

Soothing Pear Paradise (Serves 1) 33

Gentle Green Goddess (Serves 1) 33

Berry Boost (Serves 1)... 34

Tropical Tango (Serves 1)... 35

Creamy Carrot Calmer (Serves 1)............................. 35

Sunshine Citrus Smoothie (Serves 1) 36

Minty Melon Magic (Serves 1)................................. 37

Spiced Apple Delight (Serves 1)............................... 37

Berry Blast (Serves 1)... 38

Tropical Breeze (Serves 1)................................. 39

Green Goddess (Serves 1)................................. 39

Pear Paradise (Serves 1)................................. 40

Calming Citrus Cooler (Serves 1 40

Tropical Dream (Serves 1)................................. 41

Berry Banana Bliss (Serves 1) 42

Chapter 4:.. 44

Energizing Smoothies for Overall Digestive Wellness and
Immune Boost 44

Berry Chia Boost: 44

Tropical Sunshine Smoothie:..................... 44

Green Power Punch: 45

Citrus Immunity Smoothie......................... 45

Spiced Berry Blast 46

Creamy Carrot Delight:............................. 46

Tropical Green Dream: 46

Berry Banana Blitz:.................................... 47

Apple Berry Blast: 47

Creamy Pear Paradise: 48

Tropical Tango Twist: 48

Green Veggie Powerhouse: 48

Citrus Sunshine Smoothie: 49

Berry Protein Blast: 49

Creamy Apple Delight 49

Tropical Green Refresher 50

Spiced Carrot & Pear Power: 50

Berrylicious Energy Boost: 51

Tropical Green Immunity: 51

Chapter 5: 54

Creative Smoothie Variations and Customization Tips 54

5.1 Adding Protein Powders and Healthy Fats 54

5.2 Incorporating Seasonal Fruits and Vegetables: 55

Summer Sunshine Smoothie: 55

Winter Citrus Blast: 56

5.3 Adapting Recipes for Individual Preferences and Dietary Needs: 56

Chapter 6: 60

Beyond the Smoothie: Additional Dietary Strategies for
Optimal Gut Health 60

6.1 Fiber-Rich Food Choices 60

6.2 Hydration and its Importance: 62

6.3 Managing Stress and Promoting Gut Microbiome
Balance: 63

Chapter 7 66

Frequently Asked Questions About Diverticulitis and
Smoothies 66

7.1 Can Smoothies Completely Replace Meals? 66

7.2 What Ingredients Should I Avoid? 68

7.3 When to Seek Medical Attention: 69

Conclusion: Embracing a Healthier You 72

Recap and Key Takeaways: 72

Final Words from Selena Leonard: 73

BONUS 76

Diverticulitis-Friendly 7-Day Meal Plan with Step-by-
Step Smoothie Recipes 76

Breakfast: Ginger Green Glory Smoothie (Serves 1) 76

Snack: Sliced Apple with Almond Butter.............. 81

Day 2:.. 82

Breakfast: Berrylicious Relief Smoothie (Serves 1). 82

Day 3:.. 88

Breakfast: Tropical Calming Smoothie (Serves 1)... 88

Day 4:.. 94

Breakfast: Mellow Mango Magic Smoothie (Serves 1)
.... 94

Day 5:.. 101

Breakfast: Cooling Cucumber Comfort Smoothie
(Serves 1) 101

Day 6:.. 109

Breakfast: Soothing Pear Paradise Smoothie (Serves
1) 109

Day 7:.. 115

Breakfast: Gentle Green Goddess Smoothie (Serves 1)
.... 115

INTRODUCTION

Dive into Digestive Wellness: A Smooth Path to Managing Diverticulitis

Do you ever feel the discomfort of bloating, cramping, or abdominal pain, especially after eating? If so, you might be one of the millions of people worldwide affected by diverticulitis. This condition, characterized by inflammation in the pouches that develop in the lining of your colon, can significantly impact your daily life and well-being.

But fear not! This book is your empowering guide to navigating the complexities of diverticulitis and reclaiming control of your digestive health. We'll embark on a journey of understanding, exploring:

- **The intricacies of diverticulitis**: We'll delve into the causes, symptoms, and various phases of this condition, equipping you with the knowledge to manage it effectively.

- **The transformative power of smoothies**: Discover how delicious and convenient smoothies can be a valuable tool in your diverticulitis management strategy. Packed with essential nutrients and gentle on your digestive system, they offer a delightful path to optimal gut health.

Expert insights from **Dr Selena Leonard** Benefit from the combined expertise of a board-certified medical doctor specializing in internal medicine and a registered dietitian and certified nutritionist. Their combined knowledge provides a comprehensive and evidence-based approach to managing your condition.

This book is more than just a collection of recipes; it's your personalized roadmap to digestive well-being. With clear explanations, practical tips, and a treasure trove of delicious smoothie recipes, you'll gain the confidence and knowledge to manage your diverticulitis and embrace a life filled with vibrant health.

A Note from Selena Leonard:

As a fellow traveler on this path, I understand the challenges and frustrations that come with managing diverticulitis. However, I also believe in the power of knowledge, self-care, and delicious food to make a real difference. This book is my heartfelt contribution to your journey, offering support, guidance, and a touch of inspiration. Let's embark on this path together and reclaim the joy of a healthy and fulfilling life!

Chapter 1:

Demystifying Diverticulitis: Symptoms, Causes, and Management Strategies

Have you ever experienced a sudden, sharp pain in your lower left abdomen, accompanied by bloating, cramps, and constipation? If so, you might be wondering what's causing this discomfort. This chapter aims to demystify the condition known as diverticulitis, providing you with a clear understanding of its symptoms, potential causes, and various management strategies.

1.1 What is Diverticulitis?

Imagine your colon, the large intestine, as a long, hollow tube. Diverticulosis is a common condition where small pouches, called diverticula, develop on the outer wall of this tube. While these pouches themselves are usually harmless, sometimes they can become inflamed or infected, leading to a condition called diverticulitis.

1.2 Recognizing the Signs and Symptoms:

While symptoms can vary from person to person, some common signs of diverticulitis include:

> - **Abdominal pain:** This is typically the most prominent symptom, often sudden and sharp, and located in the lower left abdomen.
> - Changes in bowel habits: This can manifest as constipation, diarrhea, or both.
> - **Bloating and cramping**: These can accompany the abdominal pain and contribute to discomfort.
> - **Nausea and vomiting**: In some cases, individuals experience nausea and vomiting alongside the other symptoms.
> - **Fever and chills:** These may occur if the inflammation progresses to an infection.

It's important to note that these symptoms can be similar to other digestive issues. If you experience any of the above, seek immediate medical attention for proper diagnosis and treatment.

1.3 Understanding the Triggers and Risk Factors:

The exact cause of diverticulitis remains unclear, but several factors are believed to contribute to its development:

Low-fiber diet: A diet lacking in fiber can make it harder for stool to pass through the colon, potentially putting pressure on the diverticula and increasing the risk of inflammation.

> ➢ **Obesity:** Carrying excess weight might increase the pressure on the colon and contribute to diverticulitis risk.
> ➢ **Smoking:** Smoking is a known risk factor for inflammation throughout the body, including the colon.
> ➢ **Family history**: If a close family member has diverticulitis, you may have a higher risk.
> ➢ **Age**: Diverticulosis is more common as people age, and the risk of it progressing to diverticulitis also increases with age.

1.4 Conventional Treatment Approaches:

Depending on the severity of your diverticulitis, different treatment options may be recommended by your doctor. Some common approaches include:

> **Dietary modifications:** Increasing your fiber intake and modifying your diet to avoid certain trigger foods can help manage symptoms and prevent further flare-ups.

> **Medications:** Depending on the severity, medication like antibiotics, pain relievers, or antispasmodics might be prescribed to address infection, pain, and cramping.

> **Surgery:** In severe cases where other treatments fail or complications arise, surgery might be necessary to remove the affected portion of the colon.

Remember, this chapter provides a general overview. Always consult your doctor for personalized guidance and treatment specific to your individual needs and health condition.

By understanding the basics of *diverticulitis*, you can take proactive steps in managing your health and preventing potential complications. The following chapters will delve deeper into various management strategies, including the power of smoothies as a supportive tool in your journey towards improved gut health.

Chapter 2:

The Power of Smoothies: Benefits for Digestion and Overall Health

Beyond simply being a delicious and refreshing drink, smoothies can be a valuable tool in your diverticulitis management strategy. This chapter explores the unique advantages of smoothies, guides you in selecting suitable *Ingredients*, and offers tips for crafting balanced and flavorful blends that support your digestive health and overall well-being.

2.1 Advantages of Smoothies for Individuals with Diverticulitis:

Smoothies offer several benefits for individuals managing diverticulitis:

- ✓ **Easy to digest**: Smoothies are pre-digested due to their blended consistency, making them easier on the digestive system compared to solid foods, especially during flare-ups when chewing and swallowing can be uncomfortable.

✓ **Increased fiber intake**: By incorporating fruits, vegetables, and seeds with high fiber content, smoothies can help you meet your daily fiber requirements, which is crucial for promoting regular bowel movements and preventing constipation, a potential trigger for diverticulitis flare-ups.

✓ **Hydration support**: Smoothies contribute to your daily fluid intake, keeping you hydrated. Adequate hydration plays a vital role in softening stool and facilitating its passage through the digestive tract.

✓ **Nutrient boost:** Smoothies can be packed with essential vita

✓ mins, minerals, and antioxidants from various fruits, vegetables, and other healthy additions like yogurt or nut butters.

✓ **Versatility** and convenience: Smoothies offer endless possibilities for customization based on your preferences and dietary needs. They can be enjoyed as a quick breakfast, afternoon snack, or post-workout refreshment.

2.2 Choosing the Right Ingredients: Fiber, Nutrients, and Antioxidants:

When crafting smoothies suitable for managing diverticulitis, prioritize the following elements:

- ✓ **Fiber-rich fruits and vegetables:** Choose fruits like berries, apples, and pears, and vegetables like spinach, kale, and cooked carrots. Avoid raw vegetables during flare-ups.

- ✓ **Nutrient-rich additions**: Consider including yogurt (avoid during flare-ups) for protein and probiotics, or nut butters (avoid during flare-ups) for healthy fats and additional protein.

- ✓ **Antioxidant power**: Fruits and vegetables rich in antioxidants like berries, oranges, and leafy greens can help combat inflammation and support overall health.

2.3 Building a Balanced and Delicious Smoothie Base:

Start with a foundation of liquids that are suitable for your dietary needs:

✓ **Unsweetened almond milk:** This offers a neutral flavor and is generally well-tolerated, but feel free to explore other lactose-free options like coconut milk or oat milk.

✓ **Water:** Water is crucial for hydration and can be used as a base, especially during the recovery phase from a flare-up when fiber intake is increased.

✓ **Clear broths:** Broth can be a good option during flare-ups, providing hydration and essential electrolytes.

2.4 Tips for Perfecting Texture and Flavor:

- **Ripeness matters:** Use ripe fruits for optimal sweetness and flavor.

- Frozen versus fresh: Frozen fruits can be convenient and affordable, but fresh fruits offer a slightly different texture and flavor profile. Experiment with both options.

- **Gradual addition of frozen *Ingredients*:** Start with small amounts of frozen *Ingredients* and add more as needed to achieve your desired consistency.

- **Sweetness in moderation:** Limit added sugars and syrups. Opt for natural sweeteners like honey, maple syrup, or stevia in moderation, or explore the sweetness of ripe fruits.

- **Spices for a twist:** Experiment with spices like cinnamon, ginger, or turmeric for added flavor and potential health benefits.

- By understanding the benefits of smoothies, strategically selecting *Ingredients*, and following these basic tips, you'll be well on your way to crafting delicious and functional smoothies that contribute to your digestive health and overall well-being, complementing other management strategies for your diverticulitis.

Chapter 3:

Soothing Smoothies for Flare-Up Relief and Gut Calming

Ginger Green Glory (Serves 1)

A refreshing and mildly spicy smoothie packed with antioxidants and fiber.

Ingredients:

- 1 cup spinach
- 1/2 banana (peeled)

1/2 inch fresh ginger (peeled and chopped)

- 1/4 cup plain Greek yogurt
- 1 cup unsweetened almond milk
- Ice cubes (optional)

Instructions:

- Add all Ingredients to the blender.
- Blend until smooth and creamy.
- Add ice cubes, if desired, and blend until incorporated.

Smoothie Tip: For an extra kick of flavor, add a pinch of ground turmeric.

- Estimated Prep Time: 5 minutes
- Nutritional Values (approximate):
- Calories: 250
- Carbohydrates: 30g
- Protein: 10g
- Fiber: 4g
- Recipe 2: Berrylicious Relief (Serves 1)

A delightful and antioxidant-rich smoothie packed with the goodness of berries.

Ingredients:

- 1/2 cup frozen blueberries
- 1/2 cup frozen raspberries
- 1/4 cup chopped red apple

- 1/4 cup plain Greek yogurt
- 1 cup unsweetened almond milk
- Ice cubes (optional)

Instructions:

- Add all Ingredients to the blender.
- Blend until smooth and creamy.
- Add ice cubes, if desired, and blend until incorporated.

Smoothie Tip: For a creamier texture, use frozen bananas instead of ice cubes.

- Estimated Prep Time: 5 minutes
- Nutritional Values (approximate):
- Calories: 230
- Carbohydrates: 35g
- Protein: 8g
- Fiber: 4g

Tropical Calming (Serves 1)

A taste of the tropics with a soothing blend of papaya, pineapple, and orange.

Ingredients:

- 1/2 cup chopped papaya
- 1/4 cup chopped pineapple
- 1/4 cup orange juice (no pulp)
- 1/4 cup plain Greek yogurt
- 1 cup unsweetened almond milk
- Ice cubes (optional)

Smoothie Tip: For a touch of sweetness, add a teaspoon of honey or maple syrup.

Mellow Mango Magic (Serves 1)

A creamy and flavorful smoothie with the sweetness of mango and the benefits of spinach.

Ingredients:

- 1/2 cup chopped mango
- 1/4 cup spinach

- 1/4 cup plain Greek yogurt
- 1 cup unsweetened almond milk
- Ice cubes (optional)

Smoothie Tip: Add a pinch of ground ginger for a warming flavor.

Cooling Cucumber Comfort (Serves 1)

A refreshing and hydrating smoothie with the added benefit of cucumber's cooling properties.

Ingredients:

- 1/2 cucumber (peeled and chopped)
- 1/4 cup spinach
- 1/4 cup plain Greek yogurt
- 1 cup unsweetened almond milk
- Ice cubes (optional)

Smoothie Tip: For a touch of mint, add a few fresh mint leaves.

Soothing Pear Paradise (Serves 1)

A gentle and flavorful blend of pear and apple, perfect for sensitive stomachs.

Ingredients:

- 1/2 cup chopped pear
- 1/4 cup chopped red apple
- 1/4 cup plain Greek yogurt
- 1 cup unsweetened almond milk
- Ice cubes (optional)

Smoothie Tip: Sprinkle a pinch of ground cinnamon for extra flavor and warmth.

Gentle Green Goddess (Serves 1)

A powerhouse of greens with spinach and banana providing fiber and potassium.

Ingredients:

- 1 cup packed spinach
- 1/2 banana (peeled)
- 1/4 cup plain Greek yogurt

- 1 cup unsweetened almond milk
- Ice cubes (optional)

*Smoothie Tip:*For a touch of sweetness, add a few dates or a teaspoon of honey.

Berry Boost (Serves 1)

A quick and easy smoothie packed with the antioxidant power of mixed berries.

Ingredients:

- 1/2 cup frozen mixed berries (blueberries, raspberries, strawberries)
- 1/4 cup orange juice (no pulp)
- 1/4 cup plain Greek yogurt
- 1 cup unsweetened almond milk
- Ice cubes (optional)

*Smoothie Tip:*For an extra protein boost, add a scoop of unflavored protein powder.

Tropical Tango (Serves 1)

A vibrant and flavorful blend of pineapple, mango, and orange.

Ingredients:

- 1/2 cup chopped pineapple
- 1/4 cup chopped mango
- 1/4 cup orange juice (no pulp)
- 1/4 cup plain Greek yogurt
- 1 cup unsweetened almond milk
- Ice cubes (optional)

Smoothie Tip: Add a pinch of turmeric for its anti-inflammatory properties.

Creamy Carrot Calmer (Serves 1)

A unique and nutritious smoothie with the added benefit of cooked carrots.

Ingredients:

- 1/2 cup cooked carrot (steamed or boiled)
- 1/4 cup spinach

- 1/4 cup plain Greek yogurt
- 1 cup unsweetened almond milk
- Ice cubes (optional)

Smoothie Tip: For a hint of sweetness, add a few raisins or a date.

Sunshine Citrus Smoothie (Serves 1)

A refreshing and vitamin-packed smoothie with orange and pear.

Ingredients:

- 1/2 orange (peeled)
- 1/4 cup chopped pear
- 1/4 cup plain Greek yogurt
- 1 cup unsweetened almond milk
- Ice cubes (optional)

Smoothie Tip: For a creamier texture, use frozen pear chunks instead of fresh.

Minty Melon Magic (Serves 1)

A refreshing and hydrating smoothie with the cooling properties of melons and mint.

Ingredients:

- 1/2 cup chopped cantaloupe
- 1/4 cup chopped honeydew melon
- 1/4 cup mint leaves (fresh)
- 1/4 cup plain Greek yogurt
- 1 cup unsweetened almond milk
- Ice cubes (optional)

Smoothie Tip: Substitute mint leaves with a few basil leaves for a different flavor profile.

Spiced Apple Delight (Serves 1)

A warm and comforting smoothie with the flavors of apple and cinnamon.

Ingredients:

- 1/2 cup chopped apple
- 1/4 teaspoon ground cinnamon

- 1/4 cup plain Greek yogurt
- 1 cup unsweetened almond milk
- Ice cubes (optional)

*Smoothie Tip:*For a creamier texture, use frozen apple chunks instead of fresh.

Berry Blast (Serves 1)

A simple and satisfying smoothie packed with the goodness of frozen berries.

Ingredients:

- 1/2 cup frozen mixed berries (blueberries, raspberries, strawberries)
- 1/4 cup plain Greek yogurt
- 1 cup unsweetened almond milk
- Ice cubes (optional)

*Smoothie Tip:*For a thicker consistency, add a tablespoon of chia seeds or ground flaxseeds.

Tropical Breeze (Serves 1)

A taste of paradise with the refreshing combination of pineapple and mango.

Ingredients:

- 1/2 cup chopped pineapple
- 1/4 cup chopped mango
- 1/4 cup orange juice (no pulp)
- Ice cubes (optional)

Smoothie Tip: Sprinkle a pinch of ground ginger for a warming and anti-inflammatory kick.

Green Goddess (Serves 1)

A classic green smoothie packed with spinach and banana for fiber and potassium.

Ingredients:

- 1 cup spinach
- 1/2 banana (peeled)
- 1/4 cup plain Greek yogurt
- 1 cup unsweetened almond milk

- Ice cubes (optional)

Smoothie Tip:Add a scoop of collagen powder for additional gut health support.

Pear Paradise (Serves 1)

A gentle and flavorful blend of pear and apple, perfect for sensitive stomachs.

Ingredients:

- 1/2 cup chopped pear
- 1/4 cup chopped apple
- 1/4 cup plain Greek yogurt (or lactose-free yogurt alternative)
- 1 cup unsweetened almond milk
- Ice cubes (optional)

Smoothie Tip:For a creamier texture, use frozen pear or apple chunks.

Calming Citrus Cooler (Serves 1)

A refreshing and hydrating smoothie with the cooling properties of cucumber and mint.

Ingredients:

- 1/2 orange (peeled)
- 1/4 cup chopped cucumber
- 1/4 cup mint leaves (fresh)
- 1/4 cup plain Greek yogurt (or plant-based yogurt alternative)
- 1 cup unsweetened almond milk
- Ice cubes (optional)

Smoothie Tip: Add a squeeze of lemon juice for an extra dose of vitamin C.

Tropical Dream (Serves 1)

A taste of the tropics with a blend of pineapple, mango, and papaya.

Ingredients:

- 1/2 cup chopped pineapple
- 1/4 cup chopped mango

- 1/4 cup chopped papaya
- 1/4 cup plain Greek yogurt (or plant-based yogurt alternative)
- 1 cup unsweetened almond milk
- Ice cubes (optional)

Smoothie Tip: For a protein boost, add a scoop of unflavored protein powder.

Berry Banana Bliss (Serves 1)

A delightful and satisfying smoothie with the sweetness of berries and banana.

Ingredients:

- 1/2 cup frozen mixed berries (blueberries, raspberries, strawberries)
- 1/2 banana (peeled)
- 1/4 cup plain Greek yogurt (or plant-based yogurt alternative)
- 1 cup unsweetened almond milk
- Ice cubes (optional)

Smoothie Tip: Drizzle a tablespoon of honey or maple syrup over the top for added sweetness.

Ice cubes (optional)

Chapter 4:

Energizing Smoothies for Overall Digestive Wellness and Immune Boost

Berry Chia Boost:

- 1/2 cup frozen mixed berries (blueberries, raspberries, strawberries)
- 1/4 cup chopped banana
- 1 tablespoon chia seeds
- 1 cup unsweetened almond milk
- Ice cubes (optional)

\

Tropical Sunshine Smoothie:

- 1/2 cup chopped pineapple
- 1/4 cup chopped mango

- 1/4 cup orange juice (no pulp)
- 1 teaspoon grated ginger
- 1 cup unsweetened almond milk
- Ice cubes (optional)

Green Power Punch:

- 1 cup packed spinach
- 1/2 banana (peeled)
- 1/4 cup chopped pear
- 1 tablespoon sunflower seeds
- 1 cup unsweetened almond milk
- Ice cubes (optional)

Citrus Immunity Smoothie

- 1/2 orange (peeled)
- 1/4 cup chopped pear
- 1/4 cup chopped apple
- 1/4 lemon (peeled)
- 1 cup unsweetened almond milk
- Ice cubes (optional)

Spiced Berry Blast:

- 1/2 cup frozen mixed berries (blueberries, raspberries, strawberries)
- 1/4 teaspoon ground cinnamon
- 1/4 teaspoon ground ginger
- 1 cup unsweetened almond milk
- Ice cubes (optional)

Creamy Carrot Delight:

- 1/2 cup cooked carrot (steamed or boiled)
- 1/4 cup chopped orange
- 1/4 cup plain Greek yogurt (optional)
- 1 cup unsweetened almond milk
- Ice cubes (optional)

Tropical Green Dream:

- 1/2 cup chopped pineapple
- 1/4 cup chopped spinach
- 1/4 cup chopped mango

- 1/4 cup plain Greek yogurt (optional)
- 1 cup unsweetened almond milk
- Ice cubes (optional)

Berry Banana Blitz:

- 1/2 cup frozen mixed berries (blueberries, raspberries, strawberries)
- 1/2 banana (peeled)
- 1 tablespoon flax seeds
- 1 cup unsweetened almond milk
- Ice cubes (optional)

Apple Berry Blast:

- 1/2 cup chopped apple
- 1/2 cup frozen blueberries
- 1/4 teaspoon ground cinnamon
- 1 cup unsweetened almond milk
- Ice cubes (optional)

Creamy Pear Paradise:

- 1/2 cup chopped pear
- 1/4 cup plain Greek yogurt (optional)
- 1/4 cup unsweetened almond milk
- 1/4 cup water
- Ice cubes (optional)

Tropical Tango Twist:

- 1/2 cup chopped pineapple
- 1/4 cup chopped mango
- 1/4 cup chopped papaya
- 1/4 cup orange juice (no pulp)
- Ice cubes (optional)

Green Veggie Powerhouse:

- 1 cup packed spinach
- 1/2 cucumber (peeled and chopped)
- 1/4 cup chopped pear
- 1 tablespoon pumpkin seeds
- 1 cup unsweetened almond milk

- Ice cubes (optional)

Citrus Sunshine Smoothie:

- 1/2 orange (peeled)
- 1/4 cup chopped pineapple
- 1/4 cup chopped mango
- 1/4 teaspoon ground turmeric
- 1 cup unsweetened almond milk
- Ice cubes (optional)

Berry Protein Blast:

- 1/2 cup frozen mixed berries (blueberries, raspberries, strawberries)
- 1 scoop unflavored protein powder
- 1/4 cup unsweetened almond milk
- 1/4 cup water
- Ice cubes (optional)

Creamy Apple Delight:

- 1/2 cup chopped apple

- 1/4 cup plain Greek yogurt (optional)
- 1/4 cup unsweetened almond milk
- 1/4 cup water
- Ice cubes (optional)

Tropical Green Refresher:

- 1/2 cup chopped pineapple
- 1/4 cup chopped spinach
- 1/4 cup chopped kiwi
- 1/4 cup unsweetened almond milk

Spiced Carrot & Pear Power:

- 1/2 cup cooked carrot (steamed or boiled)
- 1/4 cup chopped pear
- 1/4 teaspoon ground ginger
- 1/4 teaspoon ground cinnamon
- 1 cup unsweetened almond milk
- Ice cubes (optional)

Berrylicious Energy Boost:

- 1/2 cup frozen mixed berries (blueberries, raspberries, strawberries)
- 1 tablespoon chia seeds
- 1 tablespoon almond butter
- 1 cup unsweetened almond milk
- Ice cubes (optional)

Tropical Green Immunity:

- 1/2 cup chopped pineapple
- 1/4 cup chopped spinach
- 1/4 cup chopped kiwi
- 1/4 cup orange juice (no pulp)
- Ice cubes (optional)

20. Apple & Flaxseed Delight:

- 1/2 cup chopped apple
- 1 tablespoon flax seeds
- 1/4 cup plain Greek yogurt (optional)
- 1/4 cup unsweetened almond milk
- 1/4 cup water

- Ice cubes (optional)

These are just suggestions, feel free to experiment with different combinations and adjust the quantities to your preference.

- ✓ Always consult with your doctor before starting any new dietary plan, especially if you have any underlying medical conditions.
- ✓ Enjoy these delicious and nourishing smoothies to support your digestive health and immune function.

Chapter 5:

Creative Smoothie Variations and Customization Tips

This chapter empowers you to personalize your smoothie experience and explore a world of flavor and nutrition beyond the recipes provided. Remember, all suggestions adhere to the list of Ingredients suitable for individuals with diverticulitis.

5.1 Adding Protein Powders and Healthy Fats:

Protein Powders: Enhance satiety and support muscle health by incorporating unflavored or vanilla-flavored protein powders. Start with a quarter scoop and gradually increase based on your needs and tolerance.

Healthy Fats: Include healthy fats like chia seeds, flax seeds, almond butter, or avocado (avoid during flare-ups) for added creaminess, sustained energy, and improved nutrient absorption. Start with a teaspoon and gradually increase based on preference.

5.2 Incorporating Seasonal Fruits and Vegetables:

✓ **Seasonal Fruits:** Embrace the vibrant flavors and potential health benefits of seasonal fruits. Consider berries in summer, apples and pears in fall, and citrus fruits in winter.

✓ **Seasonal Vegetables**: Experiment with incorporating seasonal vegetables like spinach year-round, cucumbers and zucchini in summer, and beets or carrots in winter. Remember to avoid raw carrots during flare-ups.

Here are some examples of seasonal variations:

Summer Sunshine Smoothie:

- 1/2 cup chopped mango
- 1/4 cup chopped cucumber
- 1/4 cup spinach
- 1/4 cup unsweetened almond milk
- Ice cubes (optional)

- Fall Harvest Delight:
- 1/2 cup chopped apple
- 1/4 cup chopped pear
- 1/4 cup chopped banana
- 1 tablespoon pumpkin seeds
- 1/4 cup unsweetened almond milk
- Ice cubes (optional)

Winter Citrus Blast:

- 1/2 orange (peeled)
- 1/4 cup chopped grapefruit (optional)
- 1/4 cup spinach
- 1/4 cup plain Greek yogurt (optional)
- Ice cubes (optional)

5.3 Adapting Recipes for Individual Preferences and Dietary Needs:

- **Sweetness**: Adjust the sweetness level to your taste by adding natural sweeteners like honey, maple syrup, or stevia in moderation.
- **Dietary Needs**: Adapt these recipes to accommodate various dietary needs. For example,

use lactose-free yogurt or plant-based milk for lactose intolerance.

- **Flavor Exploration**: Experiment with different combinations of fruits, vegetables, and spices to discover your personal favorites. Remember to prioritize Ingredients suitable for managing diverticulitis.

Chapter 6:

Beyond the Smoothie: Additional Dietary Strategies for Optimal Gut Health

While smoothies can be a valuable tool in your journey towards improved gut health, they are just one piece of the puzzle. This chapter delves deeper into essential dietary strategies that complement your smoothie routine and contribute to long-term digestive well-being, especially for individuals managing diverticulitis.

6.1 Fiber-Rich Food Choices:

Fiber plays a crucial role in gut health by:

- **Promoting regular bowel movements:** This helps prevent constipation, a potential trigger for diverticulitis flare-ups.

- **Nourishing gut bacteria**: Fiber acts as a prebiotic, feeding the beneficial bacteria that contribute to a healthy gut microbiome.

- **Adding bulk to stool:** This helps move waste through the digestive system more efficiently, reducing pressure in the colon, which may benefit individuals with diverticulosis (presence of small pouches in the colon wall).

Here are some excellent fiber-rich food choices:

- **Fruits:** Berries, apples, pears, oranges, and bananas (with skin).

- **Vegetables:** Leafy greens (spinach, kale), broccoli, carrots (cooked), Brussels sprouts, sweet potatoes.

- **Whole grains:** Quinoa, brown rice, oats, barley, whole-wheat bread and pasta.

- **Beans and legumes**: Black beans, kidney beans, lentils, chickpeas.

Increase fiber intake gradually to avoid potential discomfort.

Drink plenty of fluids alongside high-fiber foods for proper absorption.

Consult your doctor or a registered dietitian for personalized fiber intake recommendations based on your individual needs and health conditions.

6.2 Hydration and its Importance:

Adequate hydration is crucial for:

- **Softening stool**: This eases its passage through the digestive tract, reducing constipation and potential discomfort.
- **Aiding digestion:** Water helps break down food and facilitates the absorption of nutrients.
- **Maintaining gut health:** Proper hydration supports the function of the digestive system and promotes a healthy gut microbiome.

Aim to drink plenty of water throughout the day, aiming for at least eight glasses. Other hydrating options include clear broths, herbal teas, and unsweetened coconut water.

Listen to your body's thirst cues and adjust your fluid intake accordingly, especially during hot weather or physical activity.

Consult your doctor if you experience any concerns or difficulties maintaining hydration.

6.3 Managing Stress and Promoting Gut Microbiome Balance:

Chronic stress can negatively impact gut health by:

✓ **Disrupting the gut microbiome:** Stress hormones can lead to an imbalance in gut bacteria, contributing to digestive issues.

✓ **Increasing intestinal permeability:** This allows harmful substances to leak from the gut into the bloodstream, potentially triggering inflammation.

✓ Here are some tips for managing stress and promoting gut microbiome balance:

✓ **Practice relaxation techniques**: Activities like yoga, meditation, and deep breathing can help manage stress and promote gut health.

- ✓ **Prioritize sleep**: Aim for 7-8 hours of quality sleep each night, as sleep deprivation can negatively impact gut bacteria.
- ✓ **Engage in regular physical activity:** Exercise has been shown to improve gut health by reducing stress and promoting beneficial gut bacteria growth.
- ✓ **Consider probiotic supplements:** Consult your doctor or a registered dietitian to discuss if probiotic supplements could be beneficial for your specific needs.

Chapter 7

Frequently Asked Questions About Diverticulitis and Smoothies

This chapter addresses common questions individuals managing diverticulitis may have regarding smoothies and overall dietary strategies. Remember, this information cannot replace professional medical advice. Always consult with your doctor or a registered dietitian for personalized guidance.

7.1 Can Smoothies Completely Replace Meals?

While smoothies can be a convenient and nutritious addition to your diet, they typically should not completely replace meals, especially during the recovery phase from a diverticulitis flare-up. Here's why:

- ✓ **Limited Nutrients:** While smoothies can be packed with vitamins and minerals, they often lack the full spectrum of nutrients found in a balanced meal, including protein, fiber, and healthy fats. Replacing all meals with smoothies may lead to nutrient deficiencies.

✓ **Chewing and Satiety:** The physical act of chewing food plays a role in digestion and satiety (feeling full). Replacing meals with smoothies may not provide the same level of satiety, potentially leading to increased hunger and overeating later.

✓ **Blood Sugar Management**: Smoothies containing high amounts of fruit can rapidly raise blood sugar levels. Replacing meals with smoothies consistently may be problematic for individuals managing diabetes or prediabetes.

• However, smoothie enthusiasts can consider:

• **Incorporating smoothies as snacks:** Enjoy a smoothie between meals to add valuable nutrients and boost your fiber intake.

• Including healthy Ingredients: Choose whole fruits, leafy greens, protein powders, and healthy fats in your smoothies to enhance their nutritional value.

- **Complementing smoothies with solid meals:** Ensure your diet includes diverse nutrient-rich meals alongside your smoothie routine.

7.2 What Ingredients Should I Avoid?

While individual needs might vary, some Ingredients are generally not recommended for individuals managing diverticulitis, especially during flare-ups:

- **Seeds (during flare-ups):** While seeds like chia seeds and flaxseeds are generally beneficial, they can be irritating during flare-ups due to their texture.

- **Nuts (during flare-ups):** Similar to seeds, nuts can be irritating during flare-ups due to their texture. However, they can be reintroduced during the recovery phase in moderation.

- **High-fiber raw vegetables (during flare-ups):** Certain raw vegetables like broccoli, cauliflower, and raw carrots can be difficult to digest and potentially irritate the gut during flare-ups. Cooked versions of these vegetables are generally tolerated better.

- **Alcohol and caffeine:** Excessive alcohol and caffeine consumption can irritate the digestive system and may worsen symptoms during flare-ups.

- **Spicy foods:** Spicy foods can be irritating for some individuals managing diverticulitis and should be avoided during flare-ups or if they trigger discomfort.

7.3 When to Seek Medical Attention:

It is crucial to seek medical attention immediately if you experience any of the following symptoms, which can be signs of a severe diverticulitis flare-up or other medical complications:

Severe abdominal pain: This could indicate a more serious condition requiring immediate medical evaluation.

Fever: A fever, especially alongside abdominal pain, can be a sign of infection and requires medical attention.

Bleeding from the rectum: This is a serious symptom and needs immediate medical evaluation.

Persistent nausea and vomiting: If these symptoms persist or become severe, seek medical attention promptly.

Inability to tolerate fluids or food: This can indicate a complication and requires medical intervention.

Conclusion: Embracing a Healthier You

Recap and Key Takeaways:

This journey through the complexities of diverticulitis and the power of smoothies has hopefully equipped you with valuable knowledge and practical tools to navigate your path towards improved gut health. Let's revisit some key takeaways:

- ✓ **Understanding diverticulitis:** By recognizing the symptoms, potential triggers, and management strategies, you can take proactive steps to prevent flare-ups and improve your overall well-being.
- ✓ **The power of smoothies:** Smoothies, when crafted with the right Ingredients, can be a delicious and convenient way to support your digestive health by providing essential nutrients, promoting hydration, and easing digestion.
- ✓ Holistic approach: Remember, managing diverticulitis often requires a multi-faceted approach. Alongside incorporating smoothies into

your routine, prioritize a balanced diet rich in fiber, regular physical activity, and stress management techniques.

✓ Resources and Additional Information:

✓ This book serves as a starting point. To further your knowledge and explore additional resources, consider:

✓ **Consulting your doctor or a registered dietitian:** They can provide personalized guidance and recommendations tailored to your specific needs and health condition.

✓ **Reliable websites:** Look for reputable websites of organizations like the National Institutes of Health (NIH) or the Mayo Clinic for evidence-based information on diverticulitis and digestive health.

✓ **Support groups:** Connecting with others managing similar conditions can offer valuable support and encouragement.

Final Words from Selena Leonard:

My hope is that this book has empowered you to take charge of your health and embrace a life filled with vibrant well-being. Remember, you are not alone on this journey.

With knowledge, self-care, and a touch of creativity in the kitchen, you can navigate the challenges of diverticulitis and thrive with a healthy and fulfilling life.

Farewell, and best wishes on your journey towards optimal gut health!

BONUS

Diverticulitis-Friendly 7-Day Meal Plan with Step-by-Step Smoothie Recipes

Breakfast: Ginger Green Glory Smoothie (Serves 1)

A refreshing and mildly spicy smoothie packed with antioxidants and fiber.

Ingredients:

- 1 cup spinach
- 1/2 banana (peeled)
- 1/2 inch fresh ginger (peeled and chopped)
- 1/4 cup plain Greek yogurt
- 1 cup unsweetened almond milk
- Ice cubes (optional)

Instructions:

- Wash and chop the spinach.
- Peel and chop the banana and ginger.

- Add all ingredients to a blender.
- Blend until smooth and creamy.

Add ice cubes, if desired, and blend again until incorporated.

Smoothie Tip: For an extra kick of flavor, add a pinch of ground turmeric.

Estimated Prep Time: 5 minutes

Approximate Nutritional Values (per serving):

- Calories: 250
- Carbohydrates: 30g
- Protein: 10g
- Fiber: 4g
- Lunch: Grilled Chicken Breast with Brown Rice and Steamed Broccoli

Ingredients:

- 1 boneless, skinless chicken breast
- 1/2 cup uncooked brown rice
- 1 cup broccoli florets
- Olive oil (optional)

- Salt and pepper to taste

Instructions:

- **Marinate the chicken (optional):** You can marinate the chicken breast for extra flavor. Combine your desired marinade ingredients (e.g., olive oil, lemon juice, herbs, spices) in a bowl. Add the chicken and let it sit for at least 30 minutes.

- **Cook the brown rice:** Rinse the brown rice in a fine-mesh strainer. In a pot, combine the rinsed rice with 1 1/2 cups of water (or follow package instructions for water-to-rice ratio). Bring to a boil, then reduce heat, cover, and simmer for 45-50 minutes, or until cooked through and fluffy.

- **Steam the broccoli:** While the rice is cooking, fill a pot with about an inch of water. Bring the water to a boil. Place the broccoli florets in a steamer basket and set it over the boiling water. Cover the pot and steam the broccoli for 5-7 minutes, or until tender-crisp.

- **Grill the chicken:** Preheat your grill to medium-high heat (around 400°F). Brush the chicken breast with a little olive oil (optional) and season with salt and pepper. Grill the chicken for 5-7 minutes per side, or until cooked through (internal temperature should reach 165°F).

- **Assemble the meal:** Serve the cooked brown rice, steamed broccoli, and grilled chicken breast on a plate. Enjoy!

Dinner: Salmon with Roasted Sweet Potatoes and Green Beans

Ingredients:

- 1 salmon fillet (about 6 oz)
- 1 medium sweet potato, peeled and diced
- 1 cup green beans, trimmed
- Olive oil (optional)
- Salt and pepper to taste

Instructions:

- **Preheat the oven:** Preheat your oven to 400°F (200°C).

- **Prepare the vegetables:** Toss the diced sweet potato with a drizzle of olive oil (optional) and season with salt and pepper. Spread the sweet potato cubes on a baking sheet. Wash and trim the green beans.

- **Roast the vegetables:** Place the baking sheet with sweet potatoes in the preheated oven and roast for 20-25 minutes, or until tender. Add the green beans to the baking sheet in the last 5 minutes of roasting.

- **Season the salmon:** Season the salmon fillet with salt and pepper. You can also add other seasonings of your choice, like lemon pepper or dried herbs.

- **Cook the salmon:** Heat a skillet over medium heat. Add a drizzle of olive oil (optional) to the pan. Carefully place the salmon fillet in the pan, skin-side down (if the salmon has skin). Cook for 4-5 minutes, or until the skin is golden brown and crispy. Flip the salmon and cook for an additional 3-4 minutes, or until cooked through (the flesh should be opaque and flaky).

- **Assemble the meal:** Plate the roasted sweet potatoes and green beans. Top with the cooked salmon fillet. Enjoy!

Snack: Sliced Apple with Almond Butter

Ingredients:

- 1 apple, washed and sliced
- 2 tablespoons almond butter

Instructions:

- Wash and slice the apple into thin or bite-sized pieces.
- Spread the almond butter on the apple slices, or serve them separately for dipping.

Tip: For a more decadent snack, drizzle the apple slices with a little honey or sprinkle them with cinnamon.

Day 2:

Breakfast: Berrylicious Relief Smoothie (Serves 1)

A delightful and antioxidant-rich smoothie packed with the goodness of berries.

Ingredients:

- 1/2 cup frozen blueberries
- 1/2 cup frozen raspberries
- 1/4 cup chopped red apple
- 1/4 cup plain Greek yogurt
- 1 cup unsweetened almond milk
- Ice cubes (optional)

Instructions:

- Wash and chop the red apple.
- Add all ingredients to a blender.
- Blend until smooth and creamy.
- Add ice cubes, if desired, and blend again until incorporated.

Smoothie Tip: For a creamier texture, use frozen bananas instead of ice cubes.

Estimated Prep Time: 5 minutes

Approximate Nutritional Values (per serving):

- Calories: 230
- Carbohydrates: 35g
- Protein: 8g
- Fiber: 4g
- Lunch: Tuna Salad Sandwich on Whole-Wheat Bread with Lettuce and Tomato

Ingredients:

- 2 slices whole-wheat bread
- 1 can (5 oz) canned tuna in water, drained and flaked
- 1/4 cup mayonnaise (or light mayonnaise)
- 1 tablespoon chopped celery (optional)
- 1/4 teaspoon dried dill (optional)
- Lettuce leaves, washed and dried
- 1 tomato slice, washed and sliced

Instructions:

- **Prepare the tuna salad:** In a bowl, combine the flaked tuna, mayonnaise, celery (if using), and dill (if using). Mix well until combined and spreadable.
- **Assemble the sandwich:** Spread the tuna salad evenly over one slice of whole-wheat bread. Top with lettuce and tomato slices. Place the other slice of bread on top to create a sandwich.
- **Cut and enjoy:** Cut the sandwich in half diagonally or as desired. Enjoy!

Tip: For a healthier option, use mashed avocado instead of mayonnaise in the tuna salad.

Dinner: Turkey Chili with a Side Salad

Ingredients:

For the Turkey Chili:

- 1 tablespoon olive oil

- 1 medium onion, chopped
- 1 green bell pepper, chopped
- 2 cloves garlic, minced
- 1 pound ground turkey
- 1 (15-oz) can diced tomatoes, undrained
- 1 (15-oz) can kidney beans, drained and rinsed
- 1 (15-oz) can black beans, drained and rinsed
- 1 (15-oz) can corn, drained
- 4 cups beef broth
- 2 tablespoons chili powder
- 1 teaspoon cumin
- 1/2 teaspoon smoked paprika
- Salt and pepper to taste

For the Side Salad:

Mixed greens of your choice

Optional salad toppings: cherry tomatoes, cucumber slices, shredded carrots, croutons, light salad dressing

Instructions:

For the Turkey Chili:

- Heat the olive oil in a large pot or Dutch oven over medium heat. Add the chopped onion and green bell pepper. Sauté for 5-7 minutes, or until softened.

- Add the minced garlic and cook for an additional minute, until fragrant.

- Crumble the ground turkey into the pot and cook until browned, breaking it up with a spoon as it cooks.

- Stir in the diced tomatoes, kidney beans, black beans, corn, beef broth, chili powder, cumin, smoked paprika, salt, and pepper. Bring to a boil, then reduce heat and simmer for 30 minutes, or until thickened and flavors are combined.

For the Side Salad:

- While the chili simmers, wash and prepare your desired salad greens and any chosen toppings.

- Combine the greens in a bowl and add your favorite toppings, if desired.

- Dress the salad with a light salad dressing just before serving.

Assemble and Enjoy:

Ladle a serving of turkey chili into a bowl.

Serve with the prepared side salad on the side.

Enjoy your meal!

Snack: Pear with Low-Fat Cheese

Ingredients:

- 1 ripe pear, washed and dried
- 1-2 slices low-fat cheese of your choice (e.g., cheddar, swiss, mozzarella)

Instructions:

- Wash and dry the pear.
- If desired, slice the pear into thin wedges or sticks for easier dipping.
- Cut the low-fat cheese into slices or small cubes.
- Enjoy the pear slices (or whole pear) with the cheese slices or cubes as a healthy and satisfying snack.

Tip: Drizzle the pear slices with a touch of honey or maple syrup for a touch of sweetness.

Day 3:

Breakfast: Tropical Calming Smoothie (Serves 1)

A taste of the tropics with a soothing blend of papaya, pineapple, and orange.

Nutritional Information (estimated per serving):

- Calories: 200
- Carbohydrates: 38g
- Protein: 2g
- Fiber: 3g
- Lunch: Lentil Soup with a Whole-Wheat Roll

Ingredients:

- 1 tablespoon olive oil
- 1 medium onion, chopped

- 1 carrot, chopped
- 1 celery stalk, chopped
- 2 cloves garlic, minced
- 1 cup brown lentils, rinsed
- 4 cups vegetable broth
- 1 (14.5 oz) can diced tomatoes, undrained
- 1 bay leaf
- Salt and pepper to taste
- 1 whole-wheat roll

Instructions:

- Heat the olive oil in a large pot or Dutch oven over medium heat. Add the chopped onion, carrot, and celery. Sauté for 5-7 minutes, or until softened.
- Add the minced garlic and cook for an additional minute, until fragrant.
- Stir in the rinsed lentils, vegetable broth, diced tomatoes, and bay leaf. Bring to a boil, then reduce heat, cover, and simmer for 25-30 minutes, or until the lentils are tender. Season with salt and pepper to taste.

- While the soup simmers, toast the whole-wheat roll if desired.
- Discard the bay leaf before serving. Ladle the lentil soup into a bowl and enjoy with the whole-wheat roll.

Nutritional Information (estimated per serving):

- Calories: 350
- Carbohydrates: 50g
- Protein: 18g
- Fiber: 15g
- Dinner: Chicken Stir-Fry with Brown Rice and Mixed Vegetables

Ingredients:

- 1 tablespoon cornstarch
- 2 tablespoons soy sauce
- 1 tablespoon rice vinegar
- 1 tablespoon honey
- 1/2 teaspoon ground ginger
- 1/4 teaspoon garlic powder

- 1 pound boneless, skinless chicken breast, cut into bite-sized pieces
- 1 tablespoon vegetable oil
- 1 cup broccoli florets
- 1 cup red bell pepper, sliced
- 1 cup snow peas
- 1/2 cup chopped carrots
- 1 cup cooked brown rice

Instructions:

- In a bowl, whisk together cornstarch, soy sauce, rice vinegar, honey, ginger, and garlic powder to create a stir-fry sauce.
- Marinate the chicken pieces in the sauce for at least 15 minutes.
- Heat the vegetable oil in a large skillet or wok over medium-high heat. Add the marinated chicken pieces and cook for 5-7 minutes, or until browned and cooked through.
- Add the broccoli florets, red bell pepper, snow peas, and carrots to the pan. Stir-fry for 3-5 minutes, or until the vegetables are tender-crisp.

- Serve the stir-fry over a bed of cooked brown rice.

Nutritional Information (estimated per serving):

- Calories: 450
- Carbohydrates: 50g
- Protein: 40g
- Fiber: 7g
- Snack: Handful of Mixed Nuts and Dried Cranberries

Ingredients:

- 1/4 cup unsalted mixed nuts (e.g., almonds, cashews, walnuts)
- 1/4 cup dried cranberries

Instructions:

- Combine the mixed nuts and dried cranberries in a small bowl.

Enjoy this healthy and satisfying snack as-is or portion it into small containers for on-the-go convenience.

Nutritional Information (estimated per serving):

- Calories: 180
- Carbohydrates: 15g
- Protein: 5g
- Fiber: 3g

Day 4:

Breakfast: Mellow Mango Magic Smoothie (Serves 1)

A creamy and flavorful smoothie with the sweetness of mango and the benefits of spinach.

Ingredients:

- 1/2 cup chopped mango
- 1/4 cup spinach
- 1/4 cup plain Greek yogurt
- 1 cup unsweetened almond milk
- Ice cubes (optional)

Instructions:

- Wash and chop the spinach and mango.
- Add all ingredients to a blender.
- Blend until smooth and creamy.
- Add ice cubes, if desired, and blend again until incorporated.

Smoothie Tip: Add a pinch of ground ginger for a warming flavor.

Estimated Prep Time: 5 minutes

Approximate Nutritional Values (per serving):

- Calories: 220
- Carbohydrates: 32g
- Protein: 8g
- Fiber: 3g
- Lunch: Scrambled Eggs with Whole-Wheat Toast and Avocado Slices

  Ingredients:
- 2 eggs
- 1 tablespoon milk (optional)
- Salt and pepper to taste
- 1 slice whole-wheat bread, toasted
- 1/2 avocado, sliced

Instructions:

- **Whisk the eggs:** In a bowl, whisk together the eggs and milk (if using). Season with salt and pepper to taste.

- **Cook the eggs:** Heat a non-stick pan over medium heat. Spray the pan with cooking spray or melt a small pat of butter. Pour the egg mixture into the pan and cook, stirring constantly with a spatula, until the eggs are scrambled to your desired consistency (soft, medium, or well-done).
- **Toast the bread:** While the eggs are cooking, toast the slice of whole-wheat bread to your desired level of doneness.
- **Assemble and enjoy:** Spread the avocado slices on the toasted bread. Top with the scrambled eggs and enjoy!

Nutritional Information (estimated per serving):

- Calories: 300
- Carbohydrates: 20g
- Protein: 15g
- Fiber: 5g
- Dinner: Baked Cod with Roasted Brussels Sprouts and Quinoa

Ingredients:

- 1 cod fillet (about 6 oz)
- 1 tablespoon olive oil
- Salt and pepper to taste
- 1 cup Brussels sprouts, trimmed and halved
- 1/2 cup quinoa, rinsed
- 1 cup vegetable broth
- 1/4 cup chopped red onion (optional)
- 1 clove garlic, minced (optional)

Instructions:

- **Preheat the oven:** Preheat your oven to 400°F (200°C).
- **Prepare the cod:** Season the cod fillet with salt and pepper. Drizzle with olive oil.
- **Prepare the Brussels sprouts:** Toss the halved Brussels sprouts with a drizzle of olive oil (optional) and season with salt and pepper.
- **Roast the vegetables:** Spread the Brussels sprouts on a baking sheet. Place the baking sheet in the preheated oven and roast for 15-20 minutes, or until tender-crisp.

- **Cook the quinoa:** While the Brussels sprouts roast, cook the quinoa according to package instructions. In a saucepan, combine the rinsed quinoa with the vegetable broth. Bring to a boil, then reduce heat, cover, and simmer for 15-20 minutes, or until the quinoa is cooked through and fluffy.

- **Optional step (flavoring):** While the quinoa cooks, heat a small pan over medium heat with a drizzle of olive oil (optional). Add the chopped red onion (if using) and cook until softened. Add the minced garlic (if using) and cook for an additional minute, until fragrant. Stir this mixture into the cooked quinoa for additional flavor.

- **Bake the cod:** After the Brussels sprouts have roasted for 15 minutes, carefully remove the baking sheet from the oven. Place the seasoned cod fillet on top of the Brussels sprouts. Return the baking sheet to the oven and bake for an additional 10-12 minutes, or until the cod is cooked through (the flesh should be opaque and flaky).

- **Assemble and enjoy:** Plate the cooked quinoa, roasted Brussels sprouts, and baked cod fillet. Enjoy!

Nutritional Information (estimated per serving):

- Calories: 450
- Carbohydrates: 45g
- Protein: 35g
- Fiber: 8g
- Snack: Greek Yogurt with Berries and Chia Seeds

Ingredients:

- 1 cup plain Greek yogurt
- 1/4 cup fresh berries (e.g., blueberries, raspberries, strawberries)
- 1 tablespoon chia seeds

Instructions:

- In a bowl, combine the plain Greek yogurt, fresh berries, and chia seeds.
- Stir gently to combine and enjoy!

Nutritional Information (estimated per serving):

- Calories: 200
- Carbohydrates: 20g

Protein: 15g

Fiber: 4g

Note: Remember that these are estimated nutritional values and may vary depending on the specific ingredients and brands you use.

Day 5:

Breakfast: Cooling Cucumber Comfort Smoothie (Serves 1)

A refreshing and hydrating smoothie with the added benefit of cucumber's cooling properties.

Ingredients:

- 1/2 cucumber (peeled and chopped)
- 1/4 cup spinach
- 1/4 cup plain Greek yogurt
- 1 cup unsweetened almond milk
- Ice cubes (optional)

Instructions:

- Wash and chop the spinach and cucumber.
- Peel and chop the cucumber (optional, for a smoother texture).
- Add all ingredients to a blender.
- Blend until smooth and creamy.

- Add ice cubes, if desired, and blend again until incorporated.

  Smoothie Tip: For a touch of mint, add a few fresh mint leaves.

  Estimated Prep Time: 5 minutes

  Approximate Nutritional Values (per serving):

- Calories: 180
- Carbohydrates: 18g
- Protein: 8g
- Fiber: 2g
- **Lunch:** Chicken Caesar salad with whole-wheat croutons and light dressing
- **Dinner:** Vegetarian chili with a side of brown rice
- **Snack:** Cottage cheese with pineapple chunks
- Lunch: Chicken Caesar Salad with Whole-Wheat Croutons and Light Dressing

  Ingredients:

- **For the Salad:**
- 2 cups romaine lettuce, washed and torn
- 1 boneless, skinless chicken breast, cooked, grilled, or poached and sliced

- 1/4 cup whole-wheat croutons (store-bought or homemade)
- 2 tablespoons grated Parmesan cheese

For the Light Caesar Dressing:

- 2 tablespoons low-fat mayonnaise or plain Greek yogurt
- 1 tablespoon lemon juice
- 1/4 teaspoon Dijon mustard
- 1 clove garlic, minced
- 1/4 teaspoon anchovy paste (optional)
- Pinch of salt and black pepper

Instructions:

Prepare the dressing: In a small bowl, whisk together the mayonnaise or yogurt, lemon juice, Dijon mustard, minced garlic, anchovy paste (if using), salt, and pepper until well combined.

Assemble the salad: In a large bowl, combine the romaine lettuce, sliced chicken, whole-wheat croutons, and Parmesan cheese.

Drizzle the light Caesar dressing over the salad and toss to coat.

Enjoy!

Nutritional Information (estimated per serving):

- Calories: 400
- Carbohydrates: 25g
- Protein: 35g
- Fiber: 4g

Tip: For a vegetarian option, omit the chicken and add additional chopped vegetables like cucumber or cherry tomatoes.

Dinner: Vegetarian Chili with a Side of Brown Rice

Ingredients:

For the Vegetarian Chili:

- 1 tablespoon olive oil
- 1 medium onion, chopped
- 1 green bell pepper, chopped
- 2 cloves garlic, minced

- 1 (15-oz) can diced tomatoes, undrained
- 1 (15-oz) can kidney beans, drained and rinsed
- 1 (15-oz) can black beans, drained and rinsed
- 1 (15-oz) can corn, drained
- 4 cups vegetable broth
- 1 tablespoon chili powder
- 1 teaspoon cumin
- 1/2 teaspoon smoked paprika
- Salt and pepper to taste

For the Brown Rice:

- 1/2 cup uncooked brown rice
- 1 cup water (or follow package instructions for water-to-rice ratio)

Instructions:

For the Vegetarian Chili:

- Heat the olive oil in a large pot or Dutch oven over medium heat. Add the chopped onion and green bell pepper. Sauté for 5-7 minutes, or until softened.

- Add the minced garlic and cook for an additional minute, until fragrant.
- Stir in the diced tomatoes, kidney beans, black beans, corn, vegetable broth, chili powder, cumin, smoked paprika, salt, and pepper. Bring to a boil, then reduce heat and simmer for 30 minutes, or until thickened and flavors are combined.

For the Brown Rice:

While the chili simmers, rinse the brown rice in a fine-mesh strainer. In a pot, combine the rinsed rice with 1 cup of water (or follow package instructions for water-to-rice ratio). Bring to a boil, then reduce heat, cover, and simmer for 45-50 minutes, or until cooked through and fluffy.

Assemble and Enjoy:

Ladle a serving of vegetarian chili into a bowl.

Serve with a side of the cooked brown rice.

Enjoy your meal!

Nutritional Information (estimated per serving):

- Calories: 400
- Carbohydrates: 60g
- Protein: 15g
- Fiber: 15g
- Snack: Cottage Cheese with Pineapple Chunks

Ingredients:

- 1/2 cup low-fat cottage cheese
- 1/4 cup fresh pineapple chunks

Instructions:

- In a bowl, combine the cottage cheese and pineapple chunks.
- Enjoy this refreshing and protein-rich snack!

Nutritional Information (estimated per serving):

- Calories: 120
- Carbohydrates: 15g
- Protein: 12g

Fiber: 0g

Tip: For a touch of sweetness, drizzle a little honey or maple syrup over the cottage cheese and pineapple before serving.

Day 6:

Breakfast: Soothing Pear Paradise Smoothie (Serves 1)

A gentle and flavorful blend of pear and apple, perfect for sensitive stomachs.

Ingredients:

- 1/2 cup chopped pear
- 1/4 cup chopped red apple
- 1/4 cup plain Greek yogurt (or lactose-free yogurt alternative)
- 1 cup unsweetened almond milk
- Ice cubes (optional)

Instructions:

- Wash and chop the pear and apple.
- Add all ingredients to a blender.
- Blend until smooth and creamy.
- Add ice cubes, if desired, and blend again until incorporated.

Smoothie Tip: For a creamier texture, use frozen pear or apple chunks.

Estimated Prep Time: 5 minutes

Approximate Nutritional Values (per serving):

- Calories: 210
- Carbohydrates: 30g
- Protein: 7g
- Fiber: 3g
- Lunch: Turkey and Vegetable Wrap on a Whole-Wheat Tortilla

Ingredients:

- 1 whole-wheat tortilla
- 2-3 slices deli turkey breast
- 1/4 cup shredded lettuce
- 1/4 cup chopped tomato
- 1/4 cup chopped cucumber (optional)
- 1 tablespoon hummus (optional)
- Salt and pepper to taste

Instructions:

- **Spread hummus (optional):** If using hummus, spread a thin layer of hummus evenly over the whole-wheat tortilla.

- **Layer the ingredients:** Place the sliced turkey breast, shredded lettuce, chopped tomato, and any optional chopped vegetables (e.g., cucumber) on the tortilla.

- **Season and roll:** Season with salt and pepper to taste. Fold the bottom edge of the tortilla up over the filling. Fold in the sides of the tortilla and roll tightly from the bottom edge to the top edge to create a wrap.

- **Cut and enjoy:** Cut the wrap in half diagonally, if desired, and enjoy!

Nutritional Information (estimated per serving):

- Calories: 300
- Carbohydrates: 30g
- Protein: 20g
- Fiber: 4g
- **Tip:** You can customize this wrap with your favorite vegetables and spreads. Some other options

include shredded carrots, bell peppers, avocado slices, or light mayo.

- Dinner: Beef Stew with Whole-Wheat Bread

Ingredients:

- 1 tablespoon olive oil
- 1 pound beef stew meat, cut into bite-sized pieces
- 1 medium onion, chopped
- 1 carrot, chopped
- 1 celery stalk, chopped
- 2 cloves garlic, minced
- 1 (14.5 oz) can diced tomatoes, undrained
- 4 cups beef broth
- 2 tablespoons Worcestershire sauce
- 1 tablespoon soy sauce
- 1 teaspoon dried thyme
- 1/2 teaspoon dried rosemary
- Salt and pepper to taste
- 2 slices whole-wheat bread, toasted (optional)

Instructions:

- Heat the olive oil in a large Dutch oven or pot over medium-high heat. Sear the beef stew meat on all sides until browned.
- Add the chopped onion, carrot, and celery to the pot. Sauté for 5-7 minutes, or until softened.
- Add the minced garlic and cook for an additional minute, until fragrant.
- Stir in the diced tomatoes, beef broth, Worcestershire sauce, soy sauce, thyme, rosemary, salt, and pepper. Bring to a boil, then reduce heat, cover, and simmer for 1-1.5 hours, or until the beef is tender and the stew has thickened.
- While the stew simmers, toast the slices of whole-wheat bread, if desired.
- Serve the beef stew hot, spooned into bowls, with a side of the toasted whole-wheat bread for dipping (optional).

Nutritional Information (estimated per serving):

- Calories: 500
- Carbohydrates: 35g
- Protein: 40g

- Fiber: 5g
- **Tip:** You can add other vegetables to the stew, such as potatoes, green beans, or corn.
- Snack: Handful of Grapes

Ingredients:

- 1 cup red or green grapes (or a mix)

Instructions:

- Wash the grapes thoroughly under running water.
- Enjoy this healthy and refreshing snack!
- **Nutritional Information (estimated per serving):**
- Calories: 60
- Carbohydrates: 15g
- Protein: 0g
- Fiber: 1g

Tip: Grapes are a good source of vitamins and antioxidants. You can also freeze them for a cold and refreshing treat.

Day 7:

Breakfast: Gentle Green Goddess Smoothie (Serves 1)

A powerhouse of greens with spinach and banana providing fiber and potassium.

Ingredients:

- 1 cup packed spinach
- 1/2 banana (peeled)
- 1/4 cup plain Greek yogurt
- 1 cup unsweetened almond milk
- Ice cubes (optional)

Instructions:

- Wash and chop the spinach.
- Peel and chop the banana.
- Add all ingredients to a blender.
- Blend until smooth and creamy.
- Add ice cubes, if desired, and blend again until incorporated.

Smoothie Tip: For a touch of sweetness, add a few dates or a teaspoon of honey.

Estimated Prep Time: 5 minutes

Approximate Nutritional Values (per serving):

- Calories: 240
- Carbohydrates: 35g
- Protein: 8g
- Fiber: 5g
- Lunch: Chicken Breast Sandwich on Whole-Wheat Bread with Avocado and Lettuce

Ingredients:

- 2 slices whole-wheat bread
- 1 boneless, skinless chicken breast, cooked, grilled, or poached and sliced
- 1/4 avocado, sliced
- 1-2 lettuce leaves, washed and dried
- Optional: Salt and pepper to taste

Instructions:

- Toast the whole-wheat bread slices to your desired level of doneness (optional).
- While the bread is toasting, prepare the other ingredients. If using, season the sliced chicken breast with salt and pepper.
- Spread half of the avocado slices on one slice of toasted bread.
- Layer the sliced chicken breast on top of the avocado.
- Top with the washed and dried lettuce leaves.
- Place the other slice of toasted bread on top to create a sandwich.
- Enjoy!

Nutritional Information (estimated per serving):

- Calories: 400
- Carbohydrates: 35g
- Protein: 30g
- Fiber: 5g
- Dinner: Shrimp Scampi with Whole-Wheat Pasta and Steamed Vegetables

Ingredients:

For the Shrimp Scampi:

- 1 tablespoon olive oil
- 2 cloves garlic, minced
- 1/4 cup dry white wine (optional)
- 1/4 cup chicken broth
- 1/4 cup lemon juice
- 1/4 teaspoon dried thyme
- Salt and pepper to taste
- 1 pound fresh or frozen shrimp, peeled and deveined (thawed if frozen)

For the Whole-Wheat Pasta:

- 1/2 cup uncooked whole-wheat pasta

Water (follow package instructions for water-to-pasta ratio)

For the Steamed Vegetables:

1 cup of your choice of vegetables (e.g., broccoli florets, asparagus spears, green beans)

Instructions:

For the Shrimp Scampi:

- Heat the olive oil in a large skillet over medium heat. Add the minced garlic and cook for about 30 seconds, until fragrant. Be careful not to burn the garlic.

- Add the white wine (if using), chicken broth, lemon juice, thyme, salt, and pepper. Bring to a simmer.

- Add the shrimp to the pan and cook for 2-3 minutes per side, or until opaque and cooked through.

For the Whole-Wheat Pasta:

While the shrimp scampi cooks, bring a pot of water to a boil. Add the uncooked whole-wheat pasta and cook according to package instructions until al dente (slightly firm to the bite).

Drain the pasta and set aside.

For the Steamed Vegetables:

While the pasta cooks, steam your chosen vegetables according to their individual needs. You can use a steamer basket set over boiling water, a microwave steamer, or another preferred method.

Assemble and Enjoy:

Divide the cooked pasta among plates.

Top with the cooked shrimp scampi and your steamed vegetables.

Enjoy!

Nutritional Information (estimated per serving):

- Calories: 500
- Carbohydrates: 50g
- Protein: 40g
- Fiber: 5g
- Snack: Yogurt Parfait with Granola and Berries
- **Ingredients:**
- 1 cup plain Greek yogurt
- 1/4 cup granola
- 1/4 cup fresh berries (e.g., blueberries, raspberries, strawberries)

Instructions:

- Layer the ingredients in a bowl or parfait glass: yogurt, granola, berries, repeat layers if desired.
- Enjoy this delicious and nutritious snack!

Nutritional Information (estimated per serving):

- Calories: 300
- Carbohydrates: 30g
- Protein: 15g
- Fiber: 5g

Tip: You can customize your yogurt parfait with your favorite toppings, such as nuts, seeds, or drizzled honey or maple syrup.